The Magic of Lemons

Using Lemons for Health and Beauty

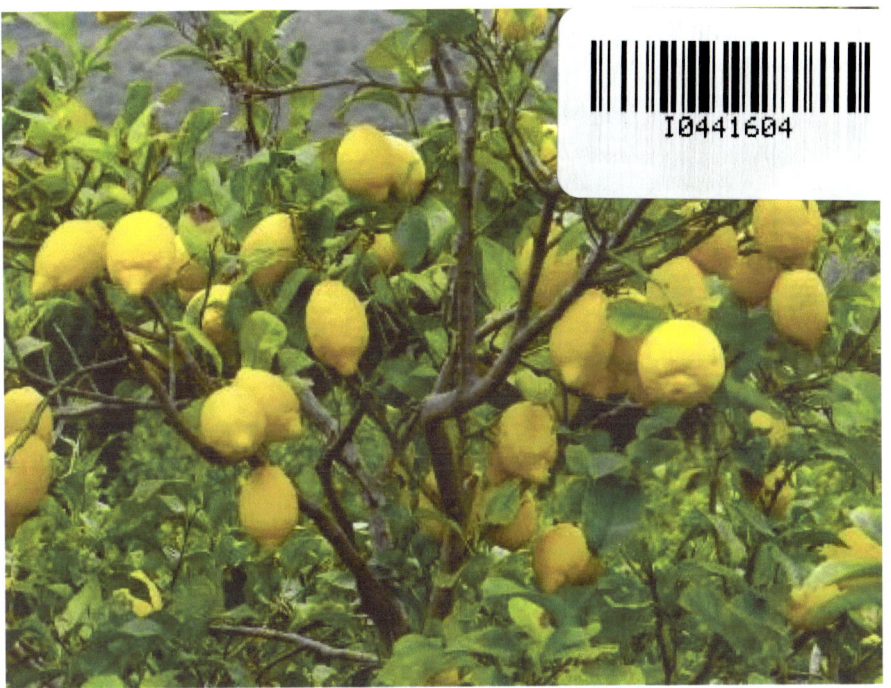

Dueep Jyot Singh

Natural Remedy Series
Mendon Cottage Books

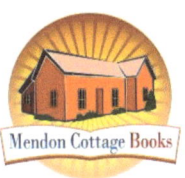

JD-Biz Publishing

Download Free Books!

http://MendonCottageBooks.com

Disclaimer

The information is this book is provided for informational purposes only. It is not intended to be used and medical advice or a substitute for proper medical treatment by a qualified health care provider. The information is believed to be accurate as presented based on research by the author.

The contents have not been evaluated by the U.S. Food and Drug Administration or any other Government or Health Organization and the contents in this book are not to be used to treat cure or prevent disease.

The author or publisher is not responsible for the use or safety of any diet, procedure or treatment mentioned in this book. The author or publisher is not responsible for errors or omissions that may exist.

Warning

The Book is for informational purposes only and before taking on any diet, treatment or medical procedure, it is recommended to consult with your primary health care provider.

Our books are available at

1. Amazon.com

2. Barnes and Noble

3. Itunes

4. Kobo

5. Smashwords

6. Google Play Books

Table of Contents

Introduction

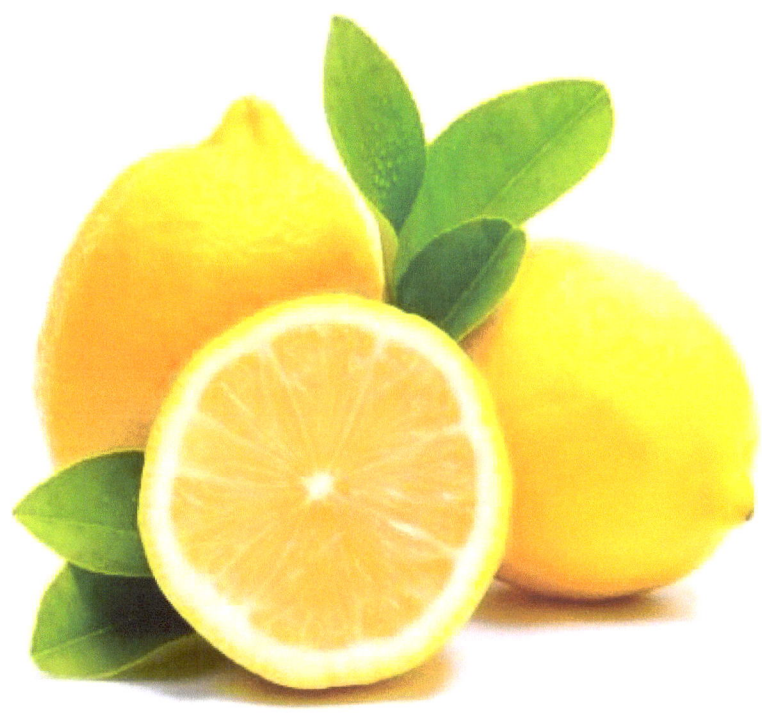

Lemon tree very pretty and the lemon's flower is sweet/but the fruit of the lemon is impossible to eat.

This song was very popular in the 60s and 70s, but the songwriter was wrong. Just not eating a lemon, because it is sour in taste, is going to prevent you from experiencing all the natural benefits of this versatile citrus fruit.

Lemons are considered to have originated in Asia, – China and Burma – from where they managed to conquer the world. Christopher Columbus brought lemon seeds back to Europe, from his travels. It thus began to be cultivated in Europe, where before it was a rarity.

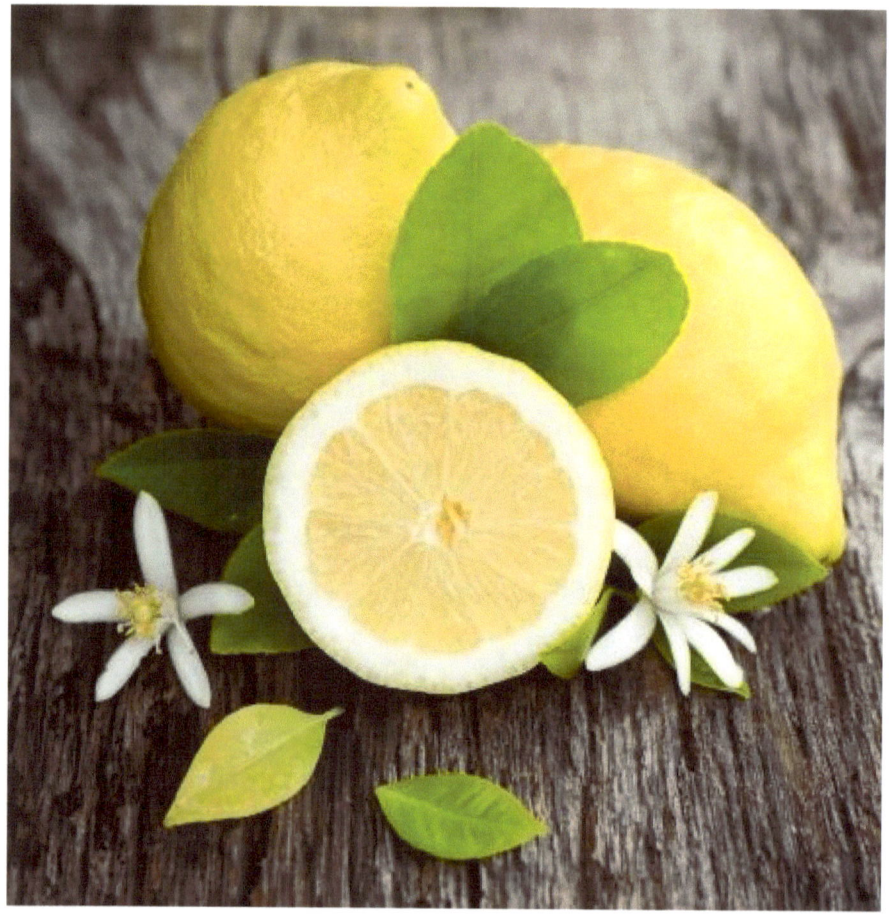

It was only in the 1740s, that people in the West began to understand that there was some power in the lemons, which prevented sailors from suffering from scurvy and beriberi. They had not heard of vitamins C at that time of course, but sailing tradition spread the word through word of mouth that whenever sailors reached some islands, they had to eat of the fruit and the grasses there. That would prevent their gums from bleeding, pain in the muscles and in the bones and make them feel healthier. These fruits were citrus fruits, including lemons.

This cause and effect apparent result made European Navies make it a rule that every ship sailing out of harbor should have a plentiful supply of lemons, green grasses and other citrus fruits to feed to the sailors and the officers, during the voyage.

However, lemons have been known since 10 A.D. in Persia, where they were used for beautifying, culinary and medical purposes. Also, their gardens used to have lemon trees, and plenty of their traditional poetry described the lemon flower along with pomegranate flowers as a symbol of beauty and grace.

The characteristic sourness of the lemon, is due to the citric acid content in it. That is why lemon juice, as well as its rind and pulp, is used in culinary preparations, all over the world. The whole of the lemon fruit can be used, with the rind ground to add a flavor to special baked dishes. Lemon juice or even the peel of the dried lemon can be used for preparing beauty products and also in natural herbal remedies.

The rind of lemon has been used since ancient times as a vermicide. This is why, after lemon juice was added to give zest to your cookery, since ancient times, the lemon rind was fed to any curious person entering the kitchen with a little bit of rock-salt. This got rid of all the intestinal parasites.

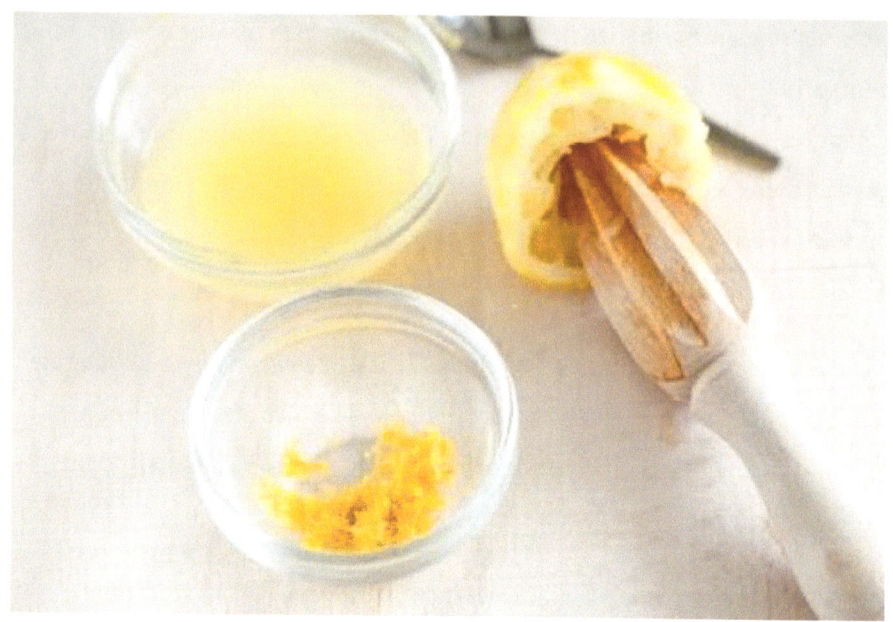

Zest, juice, and pulp – every part of the lemon is beneficial

Lemon and salt have been long in use throughout the world as natural cleansing agents. Copper cookware was traditionally cleaned by a cleansing powder made of baking soda and salt, and the scouring "pad" was a lemon. This kept the utensils squeaky clean, as well as removed any lurking vestiges of germs. Even today, in the East, if you see a silversmith working, he is going to polish a piece of silver to remove the tarnish with lemon and ashes.

Lemon has long been used as a wood polish as well as a wood cleaner. House proud ladies got rid of the accumulated grime of ages on furniture by giving it a good brisk polish with a lemon – wax polish.

The lemon as a beautifying agent has been known for centuries, when beauties in almost every civilization, including Chinese, Indian, Persian, Egyptian, Greek used citric fruits in beauty products and preparations. Nevertheless, it was not cultivated in Europe until medieval times. However, nowadays, lemons are cultivated all over the world with China, Mexico and India leading in lemon production.

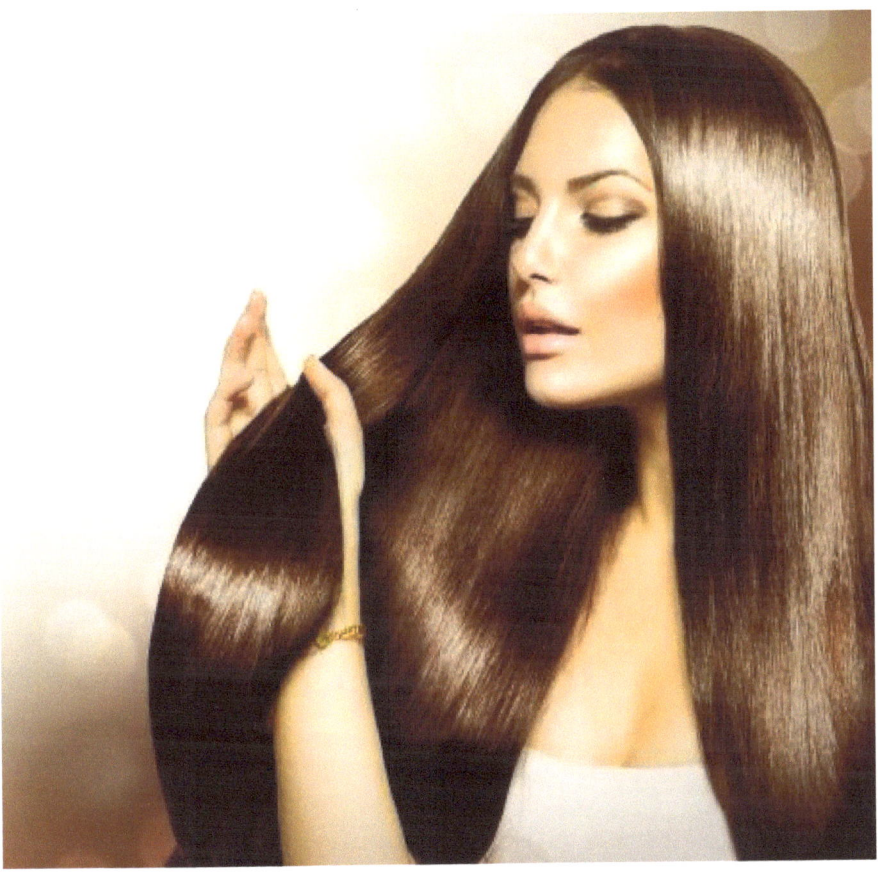

A lemon juice hair rinse is an excellent conditioner after a shampoo.

An ordinary lemon [Citrus Medica] is full of vitamin C. Along with that, you are going to find citric acid, a little bit of iron, calcium, and other minerals in this fruit. If you do not add lemons to your diet, you may suffer from scurvy, anemia, joint pain, weak teeth and bleeding gums and also asthma.

This has not been scientifically proven, but adding more lemon juice and lemons to your diet can reduce the side effects of sulphadrugs. Perhaps it is the vitamin C, which strengthens up your body in such a way that it throws off these harmful drug-induced side effects.

How to Grow a Lemon Tree

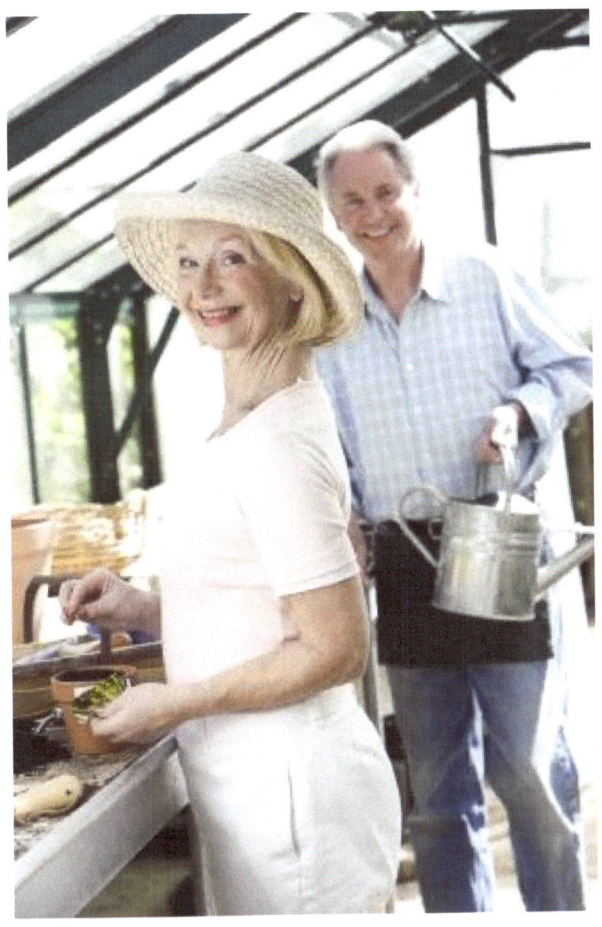

Growing your own plants from seeds can be such a relaxing activity

If life gives you lemons, make lemonade. I would go one step further, and say plant a lemon tree. You can plant lemons, in pots or in your garden.

Lemons love lot of sun, that is why they flourish so well in sunny countries, where they have an uninterrupted supply of sun and fresh air.

So if you intend to grow a lemon in a pot, which is going to be placed in your cooped up closed airless and sunless rooms, do your poor lemon a favor and decided against planting it. Instead, plant indoor flowers, which do not mind not being out in the sun. Though, I have heard there are some hybrid varieties that managed to survive indoors, especially in cold regions.

If you are living in a hot, tropical and sunny climate, this plant is going to flourish throughout the year.

The best way to grow a lemon, is to get a root cutting from a nursery. However, if you do not find a root cutting easily available in your part of the world, you may want to grow it from seed.

Now this is one experiment, which I saw an average gardener do in our neighborhood. Meyer lemons are smaller lemon plants and they can be grown in containers. But this lovely tree would be better off in your garden, with place to flourish and grow.

Our favorite gardener requested another gardener who had a lemon tree in his house to "reserve" a lemon for him. That lemon was allowed to ripen in the sun. After that, it was plucked and the seeds removed. When I asked him why he did not buy a lemon from the market, he said that he was not very sure whether it was an organic lemon or not. With organic or let us say garden grown lemons, you know that the seeds are going to germinate. You never know with possible hybrids and cultivars, where the seeds may never germinate ever,alas.

The soil in the pot, where the seedlings had to grow was well fertilized with organic fertilizer, peat and soil. Any sort of soil, which allows the absorption of water is going to do. The pot has to have an excellent drainage system. If you intend to replant the seedling into another larger pot, you can start right at the very beginning by planting it first go itself in the larger pot.

Your little lemon tree is going to settle down and put out roots in that pot. I would suggest pots which are anywhere between 16 to 22 inches in depth and up to 18 inches in diameter. But if you are getting a number of lemon seedlings prepared, you can do so with pots up to 6 inches in depth.

Your seedlings need plenty of sun, but if you are planting them in the winter, you may want a growing nursery light and a heated area. Lemon trees flourish in lands where they can get almost up to 14 hours of light. So whether it is sunlight or a grow light, Let There Be Light.

You can get excellent deals for grow lights on eBay. Prices range from USD3.25 to more, especially from China.

This particular seller

http://www.ebay.com/itm/LED-INDOOR-PLANT-GROW-LIGHT-LAMP-GROWING-PANEL-14-WATT-MICRO-GLOW-LITE-/151204820852?pt=LH_DefaultDomain_0&hash=item2334827774 is selling grow lights for USD.99.

And this one is for USD19.39.

http://www.ebay.com/itm/Miracle-LED-Indoor-Seed-Starting-Plant-Growing-Spot-Light-Grow-Bulb-Red-Blue-/111247436509?pt=US_Hydroponics&hash=item19e6dd2add

Of course, you are not going to pick out all those expensive grow lights, starting at USD149 and above, unless of course you have a nursery! So if you do not have any sun shedding its light in your particular location, try these grow lights.

Now it is time to sprout the lemon seed. Add a little water to the potting mixture, so that it is moist. Do not water log it. You do not want to drown the poor little seed, do you? You can place the soil in a bucket, add water, and mix with hand or stick until the water is absorbed in the soil, and it looks ready for planting. Put the soil back into the pot up to 2 inches from the rim.

Find a lemon seed in your lemon fruit, which looks healthy and juicy. You may either suck it or wash it, to get rid of the lemon juice or lemon pulp attached to it. Do not dry a lemon seed because that is going to finish it. I just pop the seeds in a bowl full of water, until I need to plant them.

Make a half inch deep hole in the soil. Plant the seed. Smile for a job well done. Cover it gently with soil and water with a sprinkler.

Place the pot in a sunny area, but in the shade. You do not want to give the seedlings an extra warm welcome, do you. If you are planting them in your cellar, in the winter, you need to keep the plants moist as well as warm. Make sure the temperature in your garage/cellar is pleasantly warm, and not hot. I covered the pot with a jute gunnysack, so that it did not suffer from any sort of cold draughts, due to a fall in temperature in the cellar at night.

Water regularly, and make sure that the soil never dries out. Moisture and warmth – that is necessary for your seeds to wake up and begin to take notice of their surroundings. When they germinate, which is going to be in 15 days or so, there you are, you have your seedlings ready for planting.

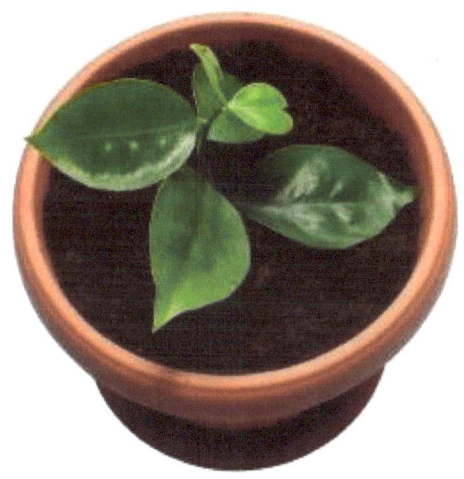

Now that the seedlings are here, it is time to plant or place them in the sun. It is going to need direct sunlight, now. Water and sunlight, and lots of loving care that is what your lemon tree needs from now on. Keep feeding it with organic compost or fertilizer just about once or twice a year, after the leaves have sprouted. I normally make a trench around my lemon plant. Then I fill it up with fertilizer or compost. After that, I turn on the garden hose. The fertilizer gets absorbed in the soil.

My lemon trees are planted in areas where there is plenty of drainage. Lemons hate having to roost in stagnant water. It is going to take anywhere between 5 to 6 years for your lemon tree to fruit, but it is going to be well worth the effort, because you have planted something for the generations to come.

Besides, it is such a nice feeling, just stepping out into your garden and plucking a ripe lemon off the tree to make into lemonade or to turn into lemon juice for culinary or beautification purposes.

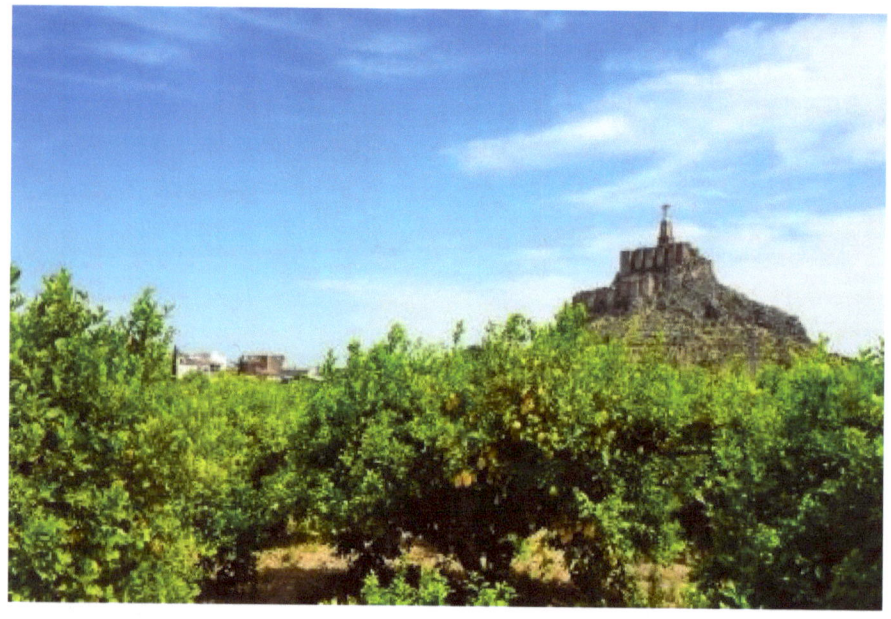

Lemon and Orange Orchard in Monteagudo Murcea, Spain

Look out for pests and brown spots. Being an organic gardener, you may use a neem oil pesticide sprayed on the plants. This is done by boiling fresh neem leaves in a bucket of water. After that, just spray with a garden sprayer. My friend in Mexico told me that her grandfather used to use tobacco water on the plants on his garden. Well, that is also a natural way in which you can get rid of pests, using tobacco, which is otherwise dangerous to your health.

Are you looking for hybrids, cultivars, grafts, or just plain lemon trees? Apart from Meyer, you can try out Rough lemon, which has more seeds and more juice, as well as a thicker skin. If you are living in Sicily, your garden has the Villafranca and the Lisbon Tree originated in Lisbon from where it reached Canada and the USA. I am sure, the original lemon plant was taken by Christobal Colon to Portugal from Spain. You can look for other tree varieties indigenous to your country, just by exploring a little.

How to Benefit from Lemons

Did you know that the best way to benefit from lemons was to never eat them raw on their own. This was something I did not know. In fact, all ancient medical books say that whenever lemons are eaten raw, they are always accompanied with rock salt/black salt and pepper. I can understand the scientific reason, now. Lemon has acid in it, and that is going to harm your intestines, if it is not neutralized with salt and pepper.

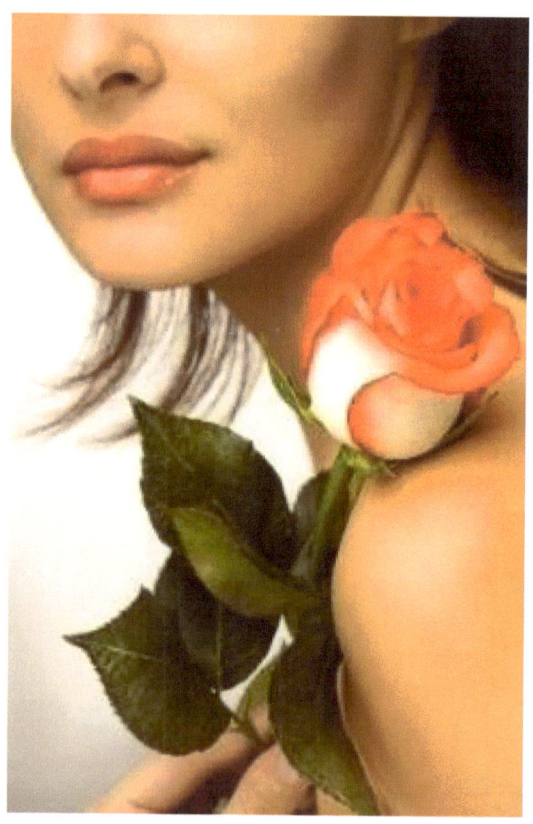

The skin we love to touch is going to keep healthy with lemon and honey.

Lemon juice on the other hand, when put in water is diluted and that is why he does not bother your digestive system much. Do not boil lemon juice. If you are drinking it in hot /warm water, you squeeze the lemon juice into the water, add sugar, honey, pepper or salt and then drink it down.

Traditional lemon squash (Nimbu pani- lit- lemon water)

8 tsp of sugar, 6 tbsp squeezed lime juice, 4 cups of water , salt to taste, crushed ice to serve.

Mix them all together and place them in the fridge.

Keep drinking as often as possible, especially in the summer or whenever you want to replenish your vitamins C, energy and water level. When you were kids, we managed about four-- 5 glasses of nimbu pani a day and never ever caught a cold in the winters or a sunstroke in the summers.

This nimbupani was also a blessing during the rare occasions when we caught a fever, because warm nimbu pani with lots of salt and pepper four times a day brought us bouncing back and in fighting trim within the week.

Apart from that, we had glowing complexions, because we did not mind rubbing the lime skins upon our cheeks to try to get rid of the sunburn!

Come to think of it, we have this habit of rubbing the skins of every single raw fruit we ate up on our faces and hands to see the effect. I must admit that apart from cooling us down and cleaning our epidermis, these fruit skins made sure that we never suffered from wrinkles or pimples.

Apart from preventing dehydration and sunstroke in the summer, lemon water is also considered to be effective in controlling HBP. People suffering from nausea are immediately given a cold dose of Nimbu paani with honey/rocksalt and pepper.

Asthma relief

Also, I found a neighbor who suffered from asthma, managing to control her breathing problems with one teaspoonful lemon juice and honey for breakfast, along with nimboo paani throughout the day.

High Blood Pressure

Remember that high blood pressure is not an ailment, it is a symptom. It is also known as the silent killer, because people suffering from high blood pressure may also be suffering from heart related diseases. Also, you never know how high blood pressure may effect one, especially if he is prone to tension, stress, strain, and other factors which could induce and aggravate HBP.

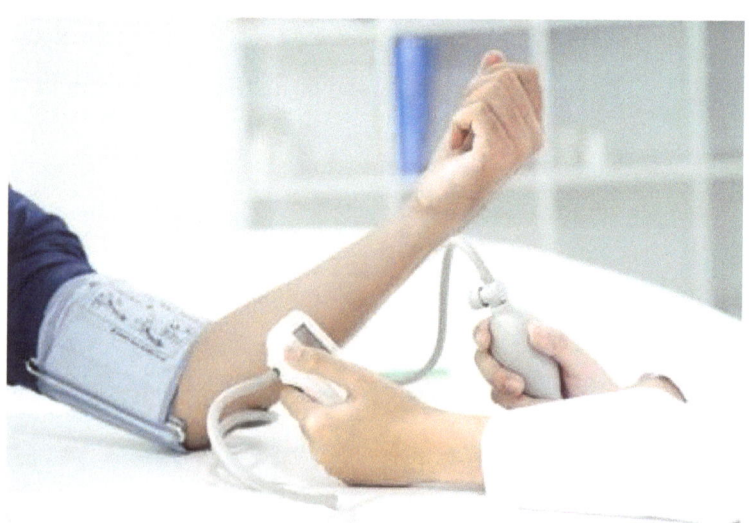

Get your blood pressure checked regularly

People eating fatty and cholesterol laden foods are definitely going to be prone to high blood pressure. Also, our sedentary lifestyles is one of the reasons why we suffer from obesity. We would rather sit in an stuffy and airless room, and do some hard mental labor than go out in the open air and do some hard physical labor.

Some of the other factors which contribute to high blood pressure, apart from a hectic lifestyle includes tobacco and alcohol intake, diabetes, gout, stress, tension, and eating an unregulated diet unsupported by exercise to burn off that extra spare tire or beer belly.

Try this way in order to manage high blood pressure. Drink 7 to 8 glasses of water every day, in which you have squeezed half a lemon. This plain lemon juice is an excellent antitoxin. It also strengthens your system.

Cantaloupe Remedy

Do you find cantaloupes or watermelons easily in your area? Well, you are lucky, because half a lemon squeezed in a glass full of fresh watermelon or cantaloupe juice, drunk once a day is going to do wonders for your HBP.

Neem Juice Remedy

If you have easy access to the neem plant, which unfortunately is indigenous in the East, but thankfully, it is being planted in many places in the West, you will need to try out this ancient natural remedy to control high blood pressure. Squeeze half a teaspoonful of juice from neem leaves. Grind fresh neem leaves in the grinder, and then add some water to this mixture. This is your neem juice, and it is a very powerful way in which you can help cure skin diseases externally. Internally, you have to be very careful about the quantity of neem juice, you ingest during the day.

So you are going to take half a teaspoonful of this juice with 2 teaspoons full of lemon juice once every day.

Believe it or not, this is going to improve your HBP problems amazingly.

Beetroot/Sugarbeet Remedy

Also, sugar beets are considered to be really good time-tested vegetables to control circulation related problems. Well, there was this time when the Greeks believed that nature had made fruits and vegetables, in the shape of organs, so that special organs could be treated by vegetables, herbs, nuts and and fruits,which were of the similar shape. So shriveled crinkled walnuts were supposed to be good for the brain, kidney beans for the kidney and so on.

Many times this guess work worked, as is in the case of sugar beets. According to Galen, beetroot juice was red in color, so it would naturally be beneficial for a human's circulatory system. So what you are going to do is drink a cup of beetroot juice with 2 teaspoons full of lemon juice, at least once a day.

Anemia Cure

Now this is a time tested lemon remedy for which I can vouch, because it worked perfectly for me. I got to know that I was anemic only when I went to a Red Cross blood donation drive, and the doctors said sorry, you cannot contribute a necessary pint, because of a low RBC count. When he saw my face blench, because I thought that I was healthy and anything low immediately gives one the feeling of doom and disaster, he said, do not worry, you just have an iron deficiency in your body. Come back after three months, after you have got the RBC count up.

Spinach Remedy

This was the remedy I used. I sipped one lemon in half a cup of spinach juice every morning for 20 days. I also increased my spinach intake in my diet. Boiled Spinach and liver fried on a griddle pan, and seasoned with lemon, Aniseed, rock salt and pepper … I boiled the spinach beforehand, so that it was already precooked, before I added the liver. Then I needed to fry both of them together, for about 5 to 6 minutes, so that both were cooked thoroughly and at the same time.

Apart from spinach I added liver to my diet. I am going to give you the liver recipe, after I have given you more anemia cures.

Carrot Juice Remedy

Drink half a cup of carrot juice in which you have squeezed the juice of one lemon, once every day for 10 days. Then go and get your blood count checked!

Pomegranate Horseradish Remedy

You may also try this pomegranate remedy. Horseradish is an integral part of the eastern diet, and that is because since ancient times, it was said that anybody who ate horseradish regularly and often never suffered from diseases of the blood. Horseradish was considered to be a blood purifier.

So take 1 tablespoon full of horseradish juice, half a cup of pomegranate juice and two teaspoonfuls lemon juice. Mix them all together, and drink sometime during the day. This is also going to increase your RBC count and get rid of the anemia problem.

Spicy Fried Liver

Tiberius Caesar suffered from anemia. The great physician Lucanus [Saint Luke] recommended that he eat three helpings of fresh bullock liver every day to get cured. Many people, including Tiberius Caesar digest liver, but if you have it spicy, at least once a day, you are going to see your RBC count growing amazingly.

1 pound lamb liver chopped in ¾ inches cubes. I am using lamb liver, because chicken liver is easily fragmented, and tends to get leathery, if it is over fried even a little bit.

One medium onion chopped finely

¼ teaspoonful each of fried cumin seeds, coriander seeds, cinnamon seeds, bishops weed, black pepper, cardamom seeds, and cayenne pepper [if you want it hot], 1/8 teaspoonful of Rosemary, thyme, Oregano, and sage. Two powdered cloves Rock salt and black salt for seasoning and taste.

You can use any spice that you like and prefer in this spice combination. There is no hard and fast rule for spices.

Remember that cinnamon, cloves and cardamoms are considered to be "heat inducing" and that is why they should be eaten in moderation in summer. Otherwise, you may find yourself suffering from skin outbreaks, prickly heat, and excessive thirst.

Make a mixture of all these items. Now you are going to marinate in liver pieces in 1 tablespoon full of this spice mixture. The rest of it can be kept in a glass bottle, to season other dishes that you make.

2 tablespoonfuls of butter to fry.

3 tablespoons Lemon juice

This is going to make two – three hungry people very happy. Fry the onion in the oil. When it is brown, add the spiced liver, which is coated with the spices, and cook at high speed for about a minute, stirring so that it does not burn. This is best prepared in a wok. When all the juices are sealed in the liver, add 1/8 teaspoonful more of the above spice mixture, for that extra zing. Continue cooking for another five minutes on high. Add the lemon after it has been cooked.

This is normally used as an accompaniment with drinks at parties, but I like to eat it spread on an egg – onion – cheese omelette, and then used as a filling in hamburger patties or in hot buttered toast sandwiches. Delicious and addictive, thanks to the lemon and black salt.

Curing a Wound Infection

This happened a couple of years ago, when I had gone exploring in the mountains. I was not near a doctor or a hospital, and somehow my traveling medical kit did not have any topical antiseptic. I hurt my arm, and did not notice it. I noticed it only a couple of days later when I found that it had been infected, had grown painful, started to itch and was oozing an infected discharge.

Honey Lemon Juice Cure

Luckily, I had a couple of lemons and a bottle of honey in my bag. I immediately made up a honey – lemon juice mixture, and bottled it. Then I assiduously began to apply that mixture on the infection, until I began to see fresh flesh and skin growing.

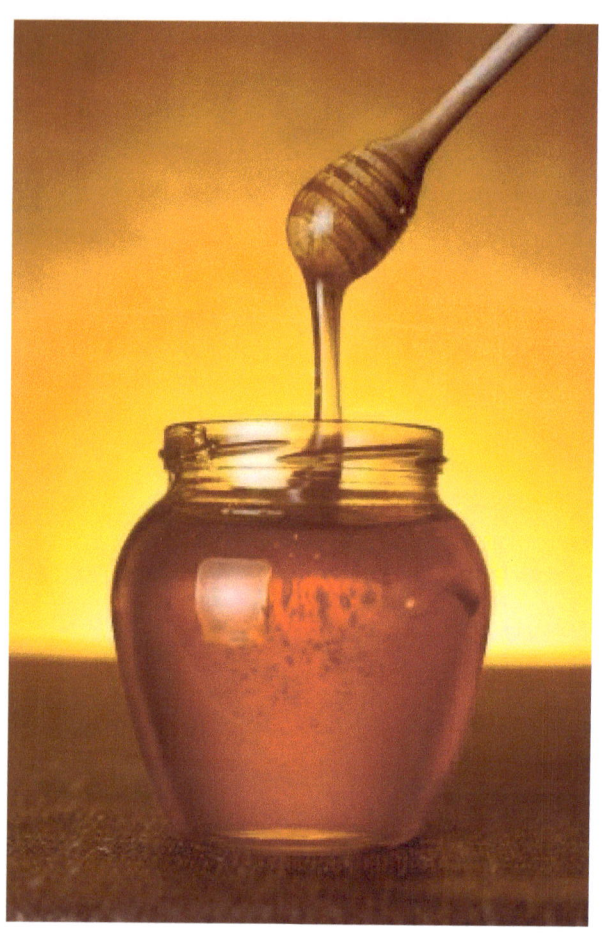

No one can beat a honey lemon combination for health and beauty.

I already knew that honey was an excellent curative to cure wounds, because it has been in use since ancient times by warriors going off to war. In fact, honey was used during the American Civil War by doctors when they did not have antibiotics or medicines around to treat the wounds of their patients. But here I was, adding lemon juice, because I did not want it to get more infected. A three-time a day application along with a cotton bandage healed that infection within 4 to 5 days. [And it was bad, believe me.] So next time you find anybody suffering from an infected wound, just dab some honey and lemon on it to heal it.

This is definitely not going to work if the wound is gangrenous. That meant that you neglected it so much, that you allowed it to be infected into the gangrene stage. This is when you need the help of experienced doctors, but for small infections, honey and lemon will save the day.

Sacred Basil Leaves Cure

If I do not have honey around, I go hunting for sacred basil. I then crush two or three leaves, mix them with lemon juice, and apply on the affected area with cotton balls.

You can also try lemon juice applied directly to the wound if you do not have honey or sacred basil around!

A friend suggested this remedy to me, and I know that it is going to work, because it has garlic in it. Garlic is the best antiseptic in your kitchen. Crush the peel of a lemon with two cloves of garlic. Now apply this paste upon that infected area. Bandage it. Renew the paste every day until the infection is cured.

Lemons are extremely versatile, so here is another remedy, which can help you, especially if you are in the kitchen and you suffer from a burn accident.

Burns Cure

The moment anybody gets burned in the kitchen, due to burning oil splashes or steam, immediately place the affected area under the running tap. This is going to cool down the affected skin. In the meantime, get out your burn cure paste from your kitchen cabinet and apply it all over the burn.

Burn Cure Paste

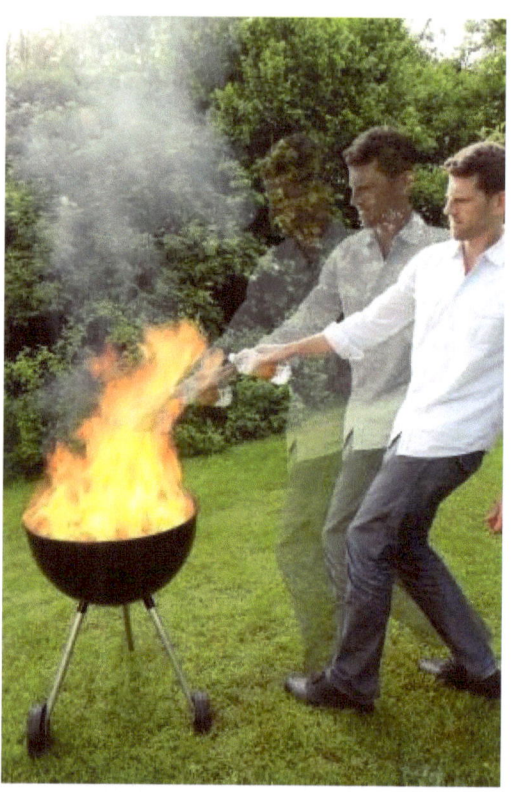

This young man will need a doctor. For other milder Burns, you can try out lemon remedies given below.

This is a burn cure paste, which is going to be made when you have plenty of lemon peels collected, and it is sunny outside. Dry the lemon peels in the shade, and in the open air. Grind them and put them in a bottle. These lemon peels in powdered form are excellent for facemasks, when mixed with dried orange peels.

You are going to take a little bit of lemon peel powder, mix it with a little bit of fresh coconut oil, and apply it all over the burn. Let it stay uncovered, because covering it does not aid in the healing process. Coconut oil is considered to be the best way in which you can heal skin naturally. I did not try olive oil, and almond oil, because I do not know about their curative properties. But this paste works really well.

Getting Rid of Burn Scars

If you find that the burn has left a scar, you can apply a paste of coconut oil, and turmeric powder to the scar. Turmeric powder is one of the best ways in which you can get rid of scars on your skin. It is an extremely useful beauty product in the East, making up natural skin creams, thanks to its antiseptic property.

If you are very badly burned, go to your doctor immediately. Do not neglect bad burns, because that may be potentially life-threatening due to infections.

Here is another burn remedy, which I find very useful.

You are going to use   rosewater here.

Rosewater

What is rosewater? Well, it is the fragrant water extracted from the petals of red roses, normally created through condensation. The side product of this extraction is rose oil. 2000 rose flowers are going to create 1 g of rose oil. That is the reason why this essential oil is extremely precious and costly.

In the same manner, if you go out to buying rosewater, in your friendly neighborhood supermarket, you are going to find it extremely costly. So it is much more sensible to make this rosewater right at home, bottle it in glass bottles, and then use it in facemasks, beauty products, food flavors, hand and face creams, and also to give that extra exotic taste to your puddings and other desserts.

How To Make Rose Water

Rosewater is normally available in markets at exorbitant prices, but in India, anybody with access to the red rose – Rosa Damascena and a little bit of time enjoys making Rosewater at home. This Rosewater is used in cosmetics, as well as in cookery to impart the flavor of the Rose to your meal or to your skin.

Ingredients needed- 1 Cup Rose petals – 12 to 14 flowers.
2 cups water
Lots of ice.
A huge cooking pan – pan number one – with lid in which another pan – pan number two – can be placed comfortably.

Rosewater is just a matter of distillation. Put a wire stand in pan number one, on which you are going to stand the other pan number two. The condensed Rosewater is going to fall into pan number two.

Place the petals at the bottom of the pan number one. Now, cover the petals with water. Place pan number two on the wire stand. Now take the lid and place it upside down on pan number one, thus effectively covering the Rose petals, pan number two and the water. The Rose water is going to condense when you place the blocks and chunks of ice on the inverted lid.

You are going to have a cupful of precious distilled Rosewater, after 25 minutes of slow steaming of the Rose petals.

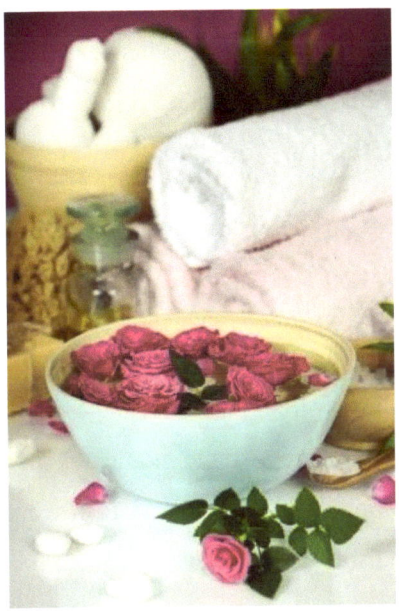

Rosewater is an important part of spas and beauty treatments

Precautions – Remember to have enough of water to cover the Rose petals. Also, it should not be of such a large quantity, that it displaces the wire stand.

This cooled water is now pure Rosewater. Pour it in a sterilized glass bottle. Use it to your heart's content. You may see a little bit of oil swimming over the surface of the water. This is Rose oil, and is even more precious. So if you used lots of petals in a larger pan, you may find even more Rose oil.

Coming back to our burn remedy –

Once you have made this rosewater, you are going to take twos tablespoons of Rosewater, 1 tablespoon of lemon juice, and 1 tablespoon full of Fullers earth. This Fullers earth is the clay, which is normally used in beauty masks. You are going to make a mixture of these items, and then apply it to the burnt area. The Rosewater cools down the skin, the Fullers Earth prevents blistering and any infection, and the lemon juice is the healing antiseptic.

Even if you do not have Rosewater around, you can always make up a paste of Fullers earth and lemon juice.

I remember an instance when my grandmother was reminiscing about the good old days, when there were no doctors, and everybody had to rely on homemade remedies and recipes. So the moment somebody broke a bone, that injured area was immediately set with slats of wood, for legs. If it was an arm injury, no wood was used.

This injury was then bandaged with a mixture of Fullers earth, ordinary lawn grass (known as Doob locally) and two eggs to make up the paste. The grass was for holding the clay together and the eggs were to bind all these materials into a covering over the wood slats for legs This bandage was then kept on for anywhere between three – six months. Nine times out of 10, the bone set by itself. This was in the 1920s – 30s, when doctors really could not be bothered to make trips to mountain areas, and one had to rely on the knowledge of the ages.

Where Do You Get Fullers Earth?

Fullers Earth is a clay-ey substance, which is easily found in beauty shops, because it goes into the making up of beauty products and facemasks.

You can easily get pure powdered Fullers earth online, but I would suggest buying it in chunks. At least then you know that you are getting pure stuff. You can grind it at home by taking a chunk, placing it on a piece of cloth, folding the piece of cloth and beating it with a heavy hammer. These smaller chunks can now be ground easily in your grinder.

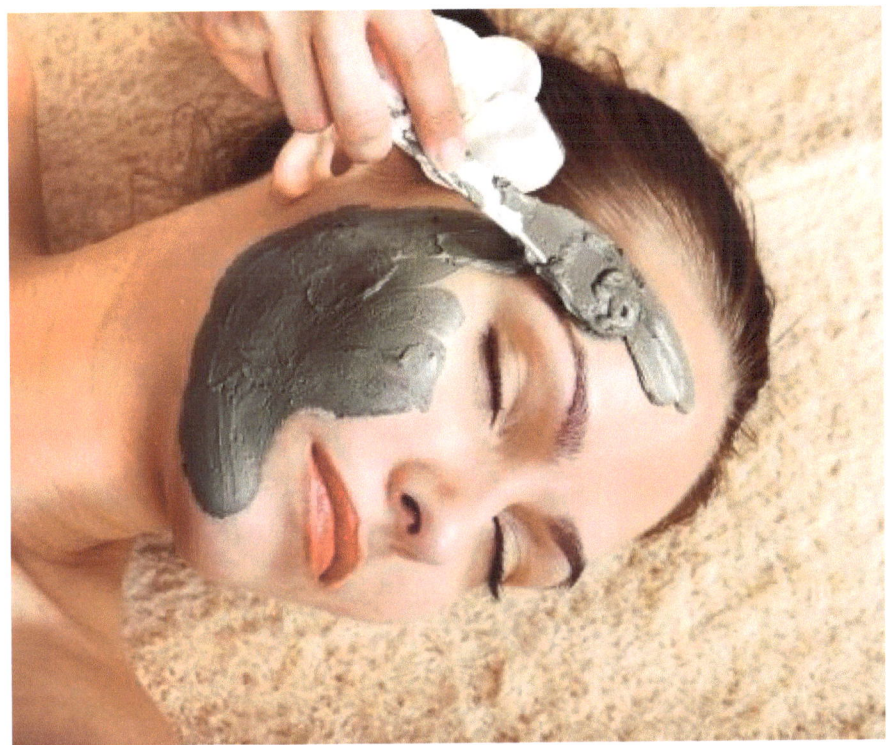

This mask consists of a Fullers Earth Base

Fullers earth and lemon juice, along with honey, and oatmeal can be the basis of your facial mask to remove the dust and grime on your skin. You can also use this combination to exfoliate your skin and leave it lovely, silky smooth and glowing. If I do not have honey around, I use cream along with rosewater, but honey is definitely the best moisturizer going.

Other Common Uses of Lemons

According to ancient treatises, the best time to eat anything with lemon, is after the sun has risen on an empty stomach, in the afternoon, or after dusk, one hour before you have your dinner. I believe these are the best times, when the tummy is ready to have more acid content added to it in the form of lemons with food following after. Use them in the afternoon by squeezing them on Salads or on your food, or just adding lemon juice to the water that you sip while eating your meals.

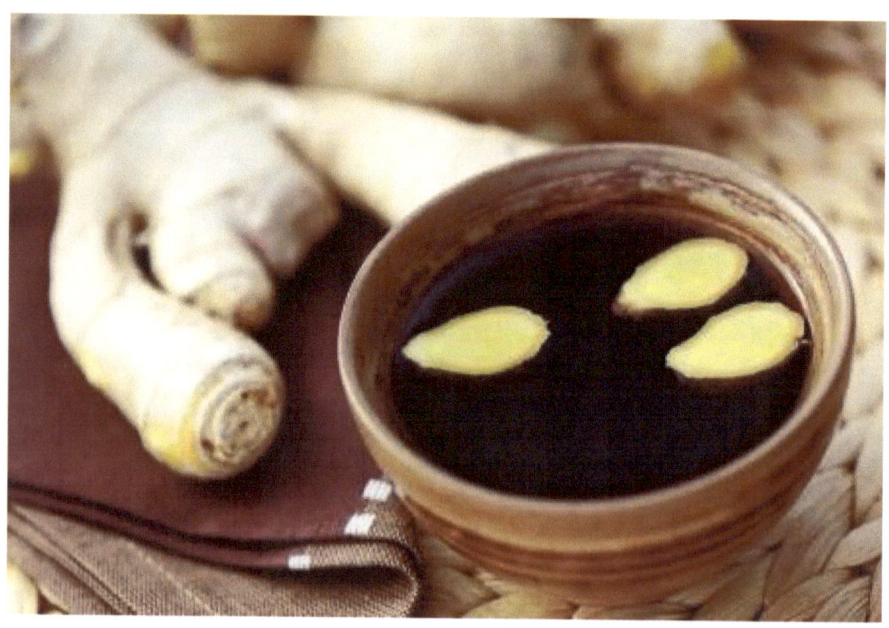

Ginger, honey, and lemon tea is delicious in the winter

There is a school of thought, which says that squeezing a lemon on cooked pulses, beans and vegetables, before eating them destroys the essential nutrients of that particular cooked dish. I beg to differ. They have already been cooked. Half of their nutrients have already been destroyed through heat. So how is a little bit of lemon juice, going to do that work, which we did in the kitchen while cooking those dishes? So I say, Enjoy lemon on your food, you are getting vitamin C.

Strain the juice, if you are going to drink it. The pulp can always be used in some other dish.

Always remember to preserve lemon juice in glass, steel, or earthenware clay containers. Never, ever keep them in aluminium, copper, iron, brass or bronze utensils.

Traditional Lemon Pickles

Here is a traditional 'limbu' pickle which is best cooked in the sun. Would you believe it, I have one of these homemade pickles, which I forgot for two years, and they aged. And I found that they are really tasty, just like aged wine and cheeses growing more delicious with the passing of time. So as long as there is plenty of salt preservative and mustard oil in them, allow them to age. I gave the glass jar another airing in the sun, and gave the pickle another lease of life for two more years.

Ingredients –

2 pounds fresh lemons
50 g rock salt.
200 g sugar/molasses
Two spoons vinegar

Pickle spices – 15 g each of cumin seed, mustard seeds, fenugreek seeds, sesame seeds, pepper, red chili powder, turmeric powder and salt. Mustard oil-To preserve the lemons.

Wash the lemons thoroughly and put them in boiling water. This is going to make them juicier. After 20 minutes, take out the lemons from the boiling water and cut them into four pieces each. You may take out the lemon juice, which we are going to use as a liquid additive during the preparation process.

Put the sugar or the jaggery together with 3 cups of water in a saucepan and allow it to cook on slow heat until it is melted completely. You may thicken this syrup if you want.

Roast all the spices then grind them into a fine paste. You may add a little bit of mustard oil during the grinding process, to make the paste more cohesive.

Now heat some of the mustard oil, and allow it to smoke. That is going to reduce the smell of the mustard oil, when you are frying the spices. Remember that frying red chili powder is going to make your kitchen a really hot place in which to remain, so make sure that your kitchen is well ventilated.

Now add the cut pieces of the lemon into this fried spice paste. Mix well. Now pour in the lemon juice and the jaggery mixture on top of this lemon – spice mixture. Place a cloth over the mouth of the glass pickle jar, and place in the sun. After two days sprinkle some more salt on and Add some more lemon juice, if you want to make it even more tasty. Mix well. After you have seasoned this lemon pickle for about 10 days, you are going to find that the skin has softened, the juice will have thickened and you can eat it, after two weeks of sun baking.

If you enter an Eastern terrace or balcony, in summer and winter, you are going to see a row of glass pickle jars, with different preserved vegetables, being prepared for the next year's eating. This is how traditional lemon pickles are made in the East.

Traditional Lemon Sherbet

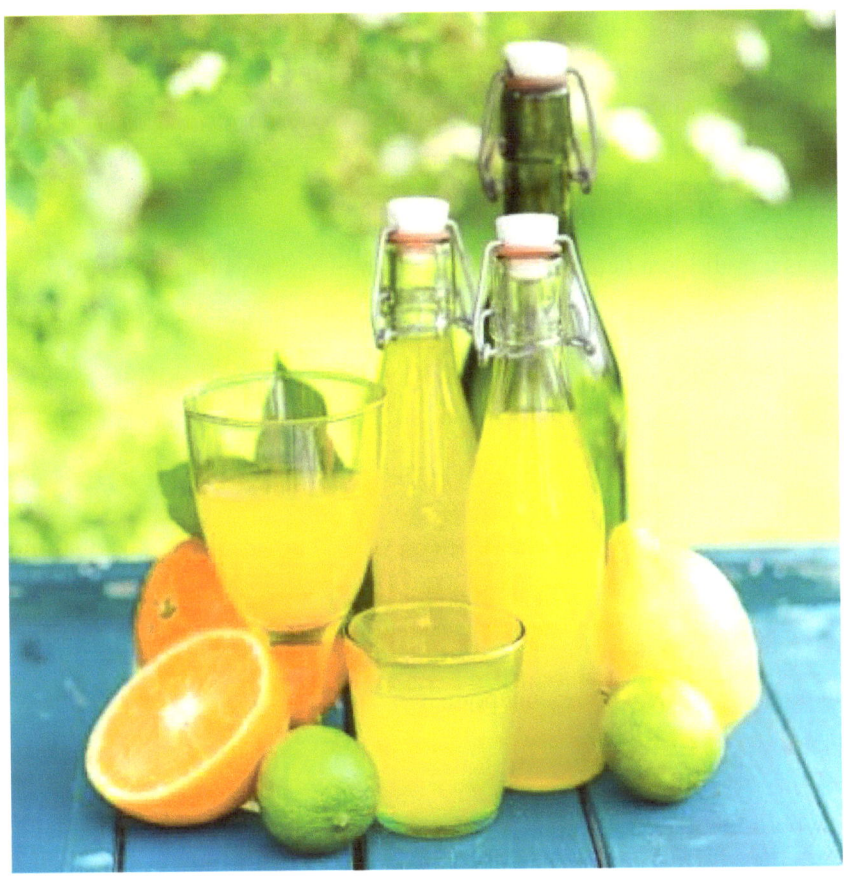

Different people have different ways of making lemon sherbet, but this is the oriental way which has passed down through centuries.

Take a kilo of sugar, and put 1 ½ kg of water in it. Set it on heat and allow the sugar to melt on a low heat. When the water is reduced to one/fourth its original quantity, add half a spoonful of alum to this mixture. Filter the mixture after it has cooled. Now you may want to add a little bit of citric acid to this mixture. Whenever you want to drink this sherbet, you just need to take a little glass of this concentrate and add it to three glasses of iced water. Stir and drink.If you want to add real lemon juice to this sherbet, take 250 g of lemon juice and add it to the cooled and filtered syrup. Mix well and bottle. This works equally well, especially if you put the bottle in the winter sun, for a little while.

Natural Bleaching Cream

This is a traditional natural bleaching cream, which was told to me by one of my beautician friends. Believe it or not, she does not use any of the beauty products marketed in the market, even though she uses them with   great success on her clients. Rather, she would prefer natural products to be applied on her skin. Talk about double standards!

So if you want to get rid of blemishes on your skin, or bleach it, add a little bit of powdered oatmeal/wheat bran/chickpea flour – also known as besan-, three pinches salt and a little bit of turmeric to 3 g lemon peel powder. Mix it in cream, or vaseline, put in a porcelain container and preserving your fridge.

Now before you go to sleep at night, you are going to rub your face, hands, arms and neck with this cleansing and bleaching mixture. Wash this off with warm water after 10 minutes.This is an amazing skin toner, cleanser and natural bleacher. You may also find the blemishes on your skin disappearing. So if you want to appear really fair, try this bleaching and moisturizing cleanser.

Lemon Cleaner

Did you notice that many of the detergents as well as cleaners have lemon extracts added to this chemical mixture? That is because these manufacturers know that lemons are the best way in which things can get really clean while leaving behind a nice lemony fragrance. So if you want to make a lemon cleaner for your utensils, just make up a mixture of salt, soda bicarbonate and some lemon juice. You may want to use the lemon peel to scrub utensils, and once they are shiny, you can always use more lemon peels.

Easy Tips

- You can get rid of odours on utensils or on your hands, by rubbing them with lemon peel.
- Added peeled and chopped apples and bananas to lemon juice. This is not going to discolor them.
- Marinating fish in lemon can reduce the fishy smell before frying.
- Add just a couple of drops of lemon juice to rice before boiling. This is going to bleach the Rice. This is also going to separate all the grains. Excellent, for when you are preparing basmati rice.
- Do you have any metal accessories in your kitchen or in your bathroom, including the sink tap? Try scrubbing them with a mixture of lemon peel and salt to bring out the shine and get rid of the grime.

- If you have delicate glass tumblers, and do not want to polish them with a rough cloth, try polishing them with lemon juice. For that, you need to fill a pan with cold water. Squeeze the juice of a lemon into the pan and place the classes in this solution. Now lift up the glasses carefully and polish gently with linen.

- Bleach your clothes without using artificial bleacher by putting the juice of one lemon in the last rinse. Now Dip the clothes in the rinse and dry in the sun. You are going to have lemon sunbleached clothes smelling fresh and crisp.

- You can remove rust stains on clothes by dipping half a lemon in some salt and rubbing the rusty area with the lemon. After that, place the cloth in the sun. This is going to make the rust stains disappear or lighten them, by making the salt and lemon bleach the cloth.

Conclusion

These are just some of the uses to which you can put lemons. In fact, lemons have unlimited uses, in cuisine, beauty remedies and natural remedies and these are just a small fraction of those uses collected in this book. Nevertheless, lemons have been used since millenniums for keeping you healthy, fit and beautiful.

 So remember that natural fruit and natural vegetables are going to be the best health giving remedies and tonics available to you. And this includes lemon juice, freshly made and sprinkled with rocksalt and pepper. This refreshing drink keeps you dehydrated, detoxifies your body and also keeps your skin glowing and youthful. It also tones of your system and prevent skin blemishes and other diseases caused by a deficiency of vitamin A and C.

Lemons and oranges are best eaten in the summer. However, if you are suffering from plenty of colds in the winter, stop eating lemons, in their of form, even though you can drink plenty of lemon juice. This is going to give you vitamins C and A, to boost up your auto immune system, and keep you healthy.

The author hopes that you found this book useful. There are more magic series available to you onAmazon, so you may want to know more about different herbs, spices, shoppers, fruit and vegetables, which keep you healthy.

Life is for living emperor size. So the next time you find yourself dehydrated due to staying out in the sun, drink lots of fresh lemon juice.

Also bleach your skin by mixing lemon juice, with salt and applying it on suntanned areas at night.

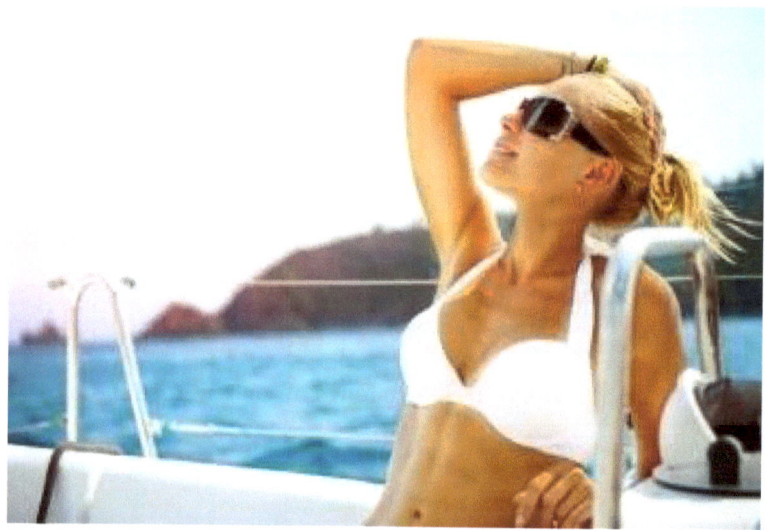

Author Bio

Dueep Jyot Singh is a Management and IT Professional who managed to gather Postgraduate qualifications in Management and English and Degrees in Science, French and Education while pursuing different enjoyable career options like being an hospital administrator, IT,SEO and HRD Database Manager/ trainer, movie scriptwriter, theatre artiste and public speaker, lecturer in French, Marketing and Advertising, ex-Editor of Hearts On Fire (now known as Solctice) Books Missouri USA, advice columnist and cartoonist, publisher and Aviation School trainer, ex- moderator on Medico.in, banker, student councilor ,travelogue writer ... among other things! One fine morning, she decided that she had enough of killing herself by Degrees and went back to her first love -- writing. It's more enjoyable! She already has 48 published academic and 14 fiction- in- different- genre books under her belt.

When she is not designing websites or making Graphic design illustrations for clients , she is busy browsing in old bookshops for antique books,-she has a mouthwatering collection of priceless First editions and rare books...including R.L. Stevenson, O.Henry, Dornford Yates, Maurice Walsh, C.N.Williamson, and the crown of her collection- Dickens "The Old Curiosity Shop," and so on... Just call her "Renaissance Woman" - collecting herbal remedies, acting like Universal Helping Hand/Agony Aunt, or escaping to her dear mountains for a bit of exploring, collecting herbs and plants and trekking.

Check out some of the other JD-Biz Publishing books

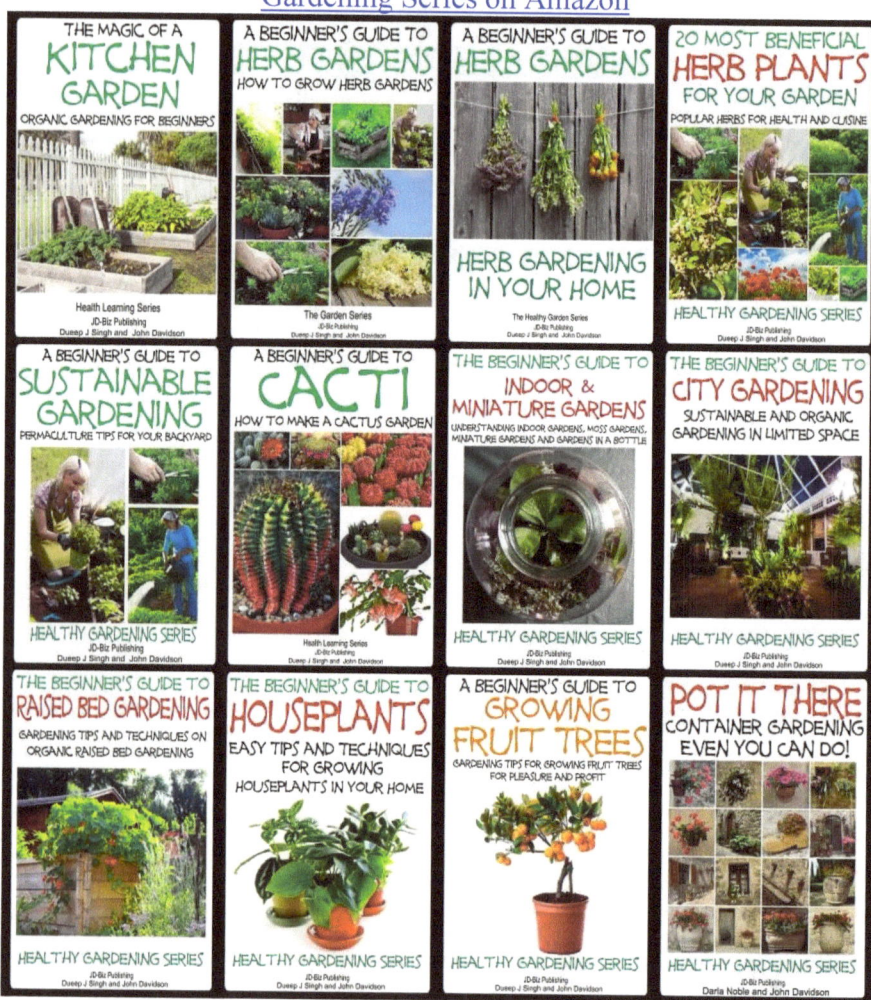

Health Learning Series

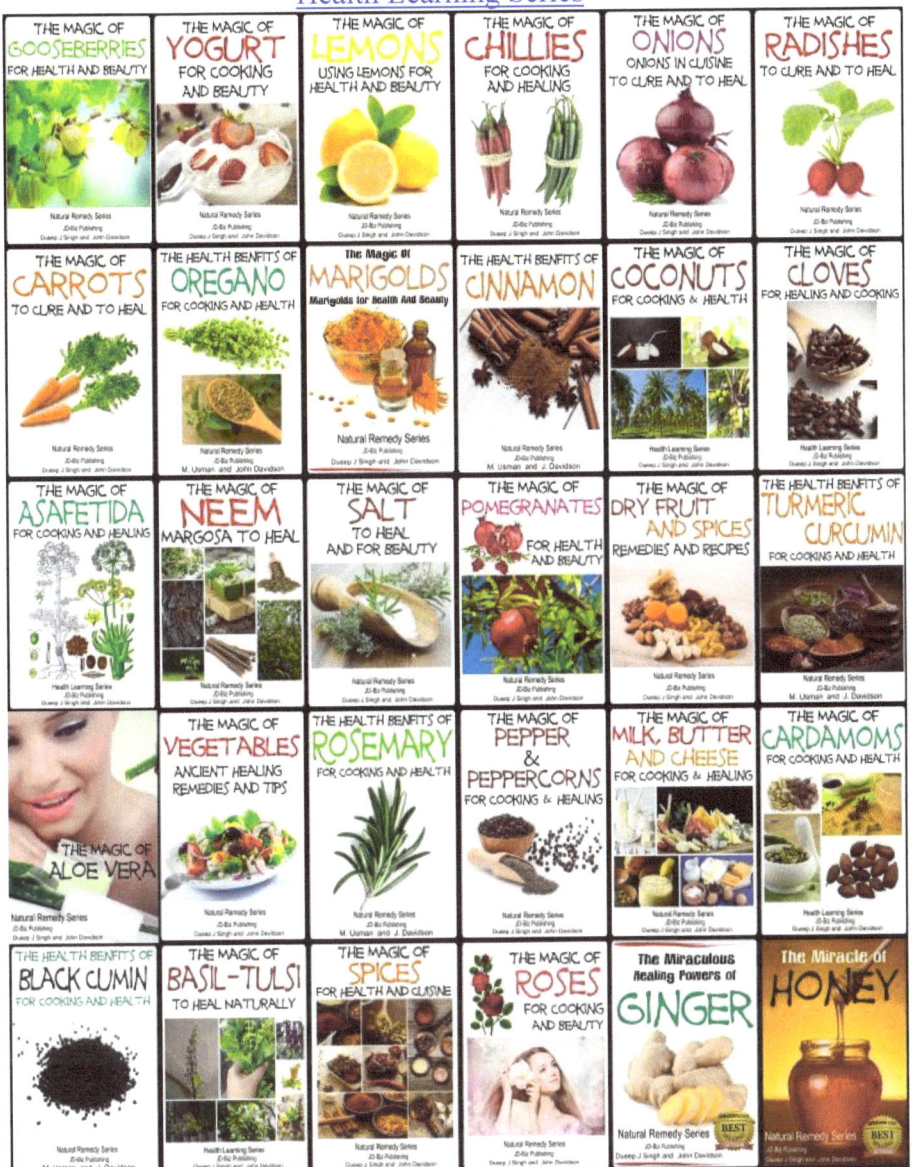

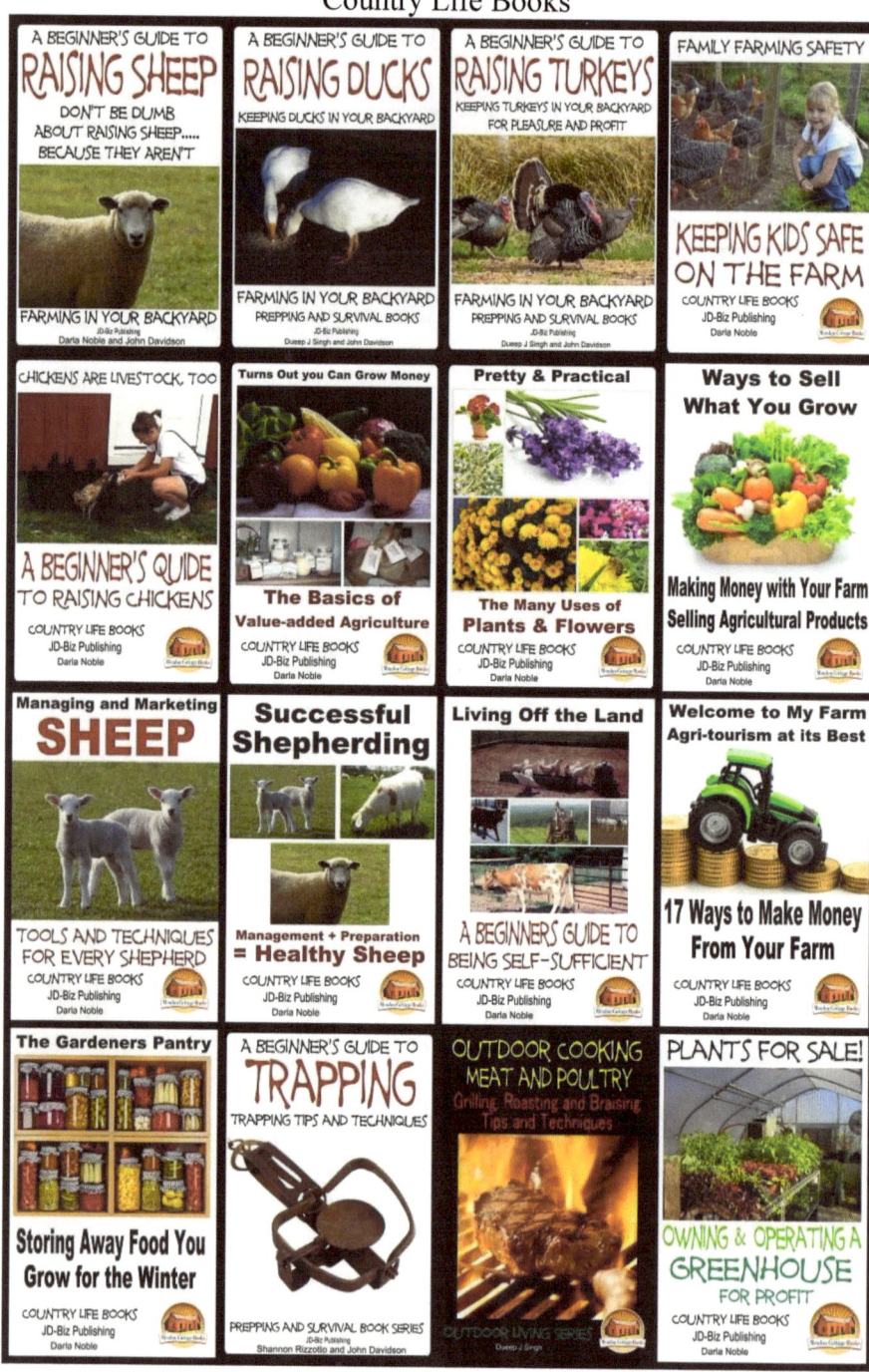

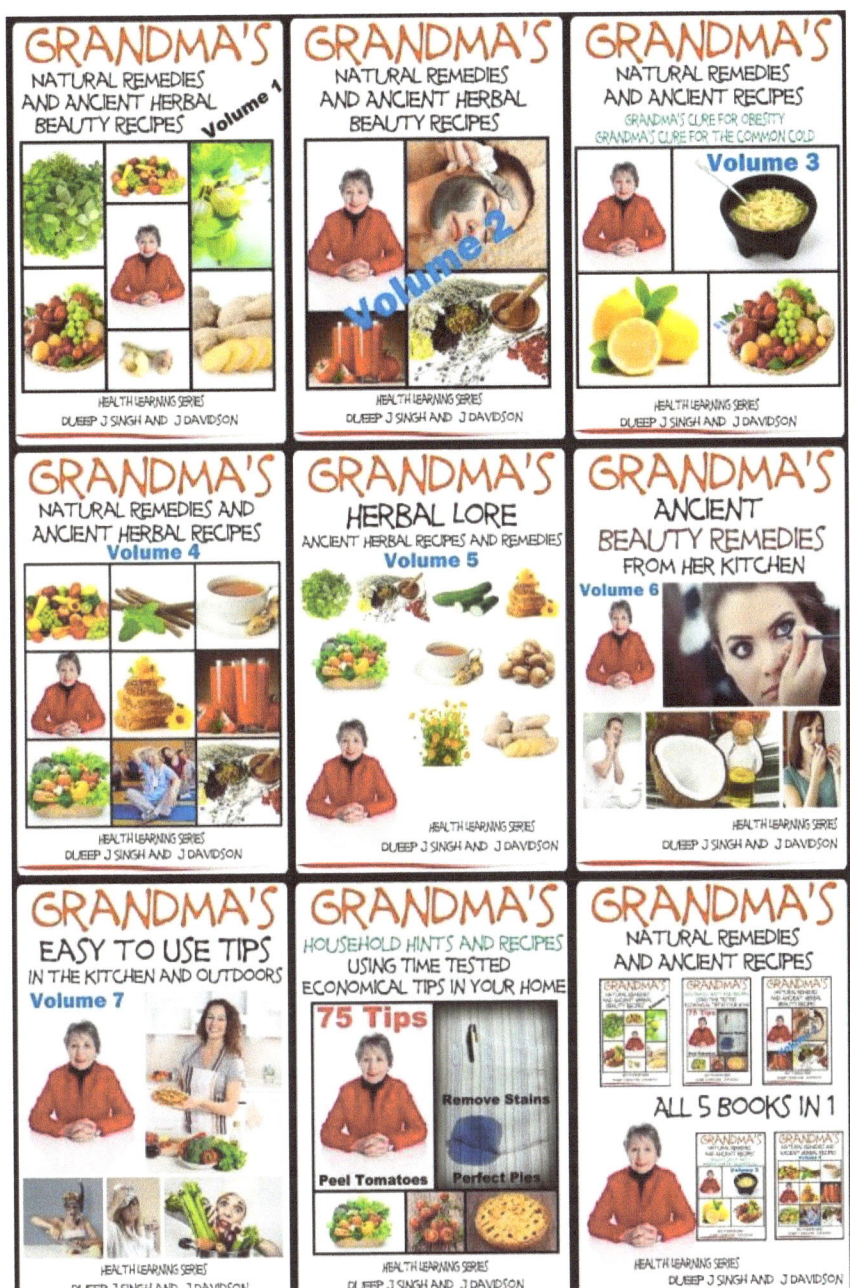

Health Learning Series

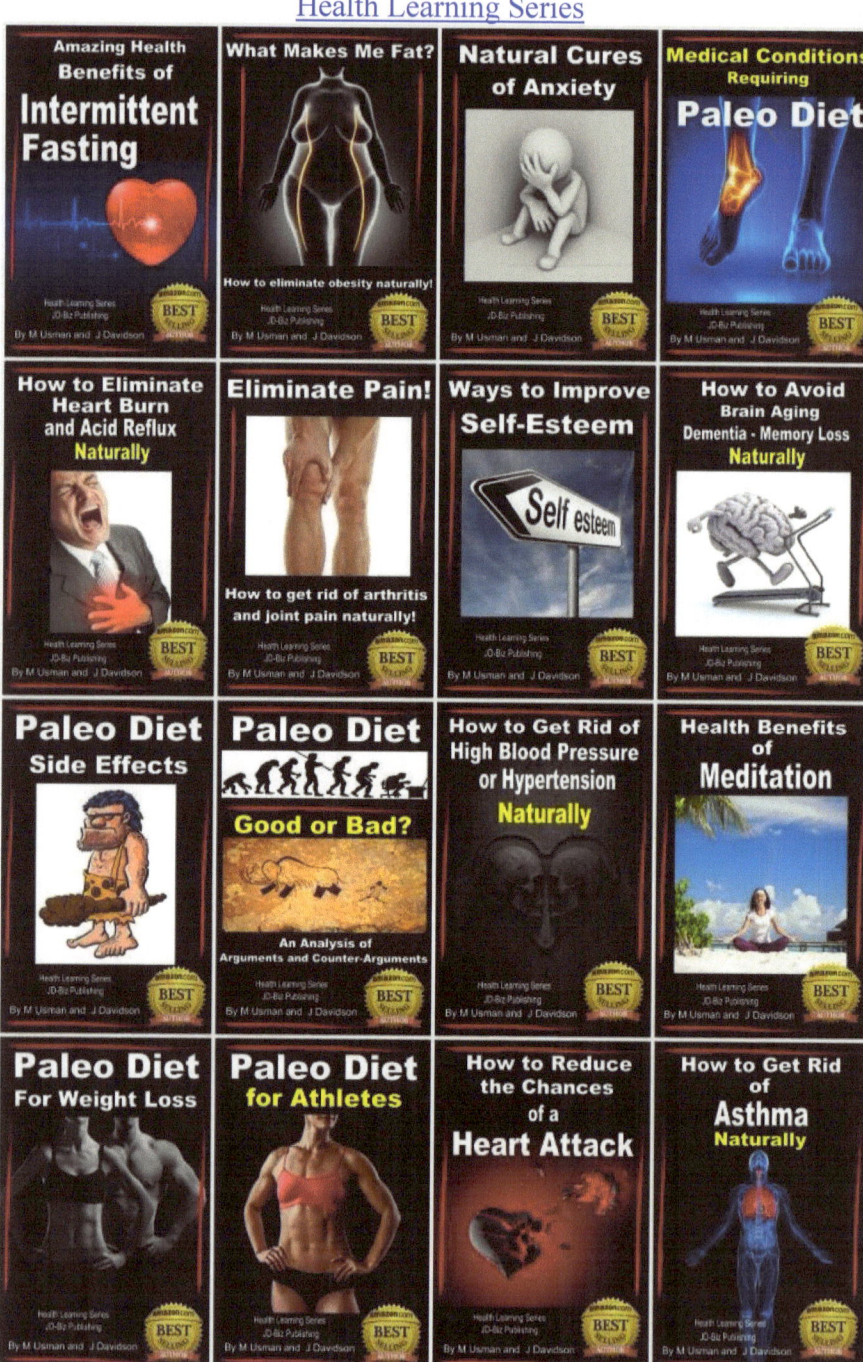

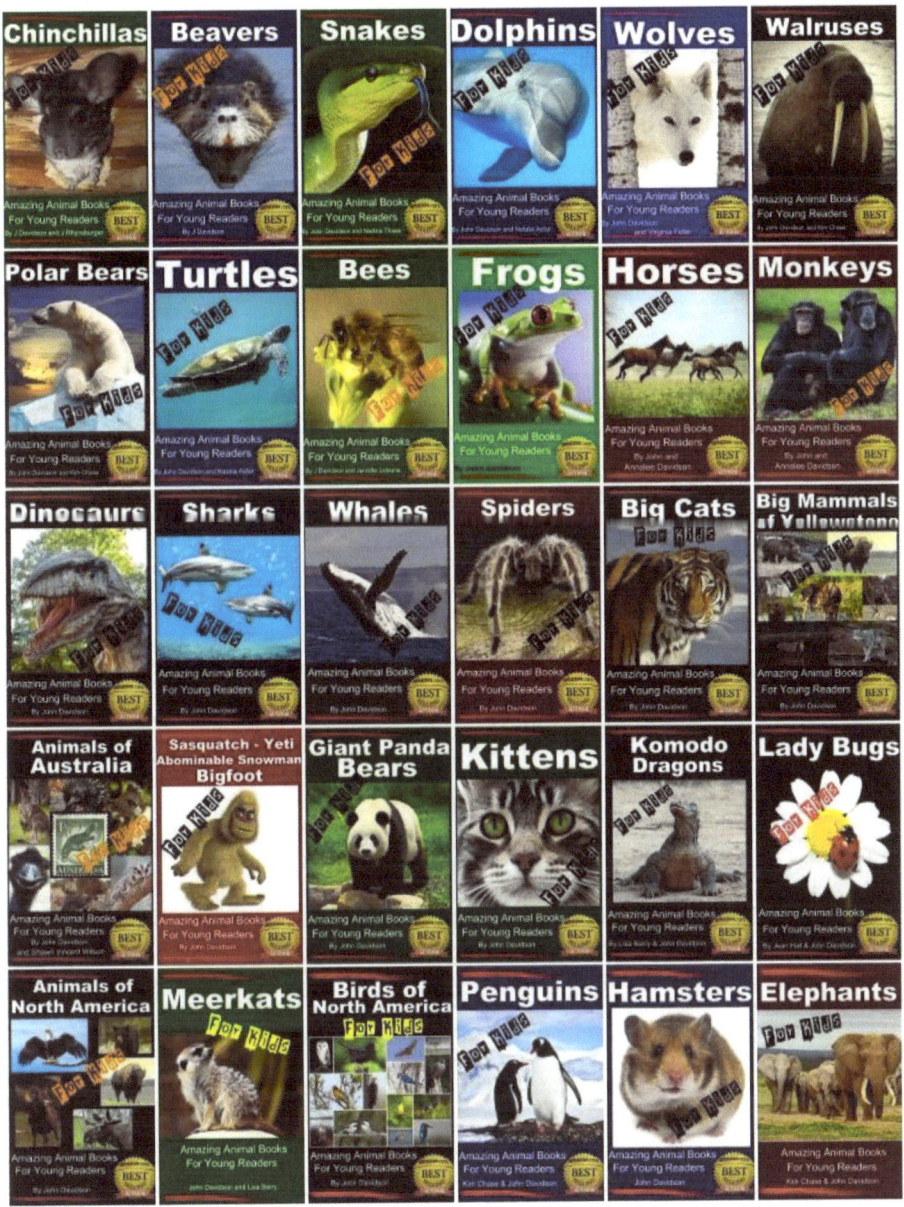

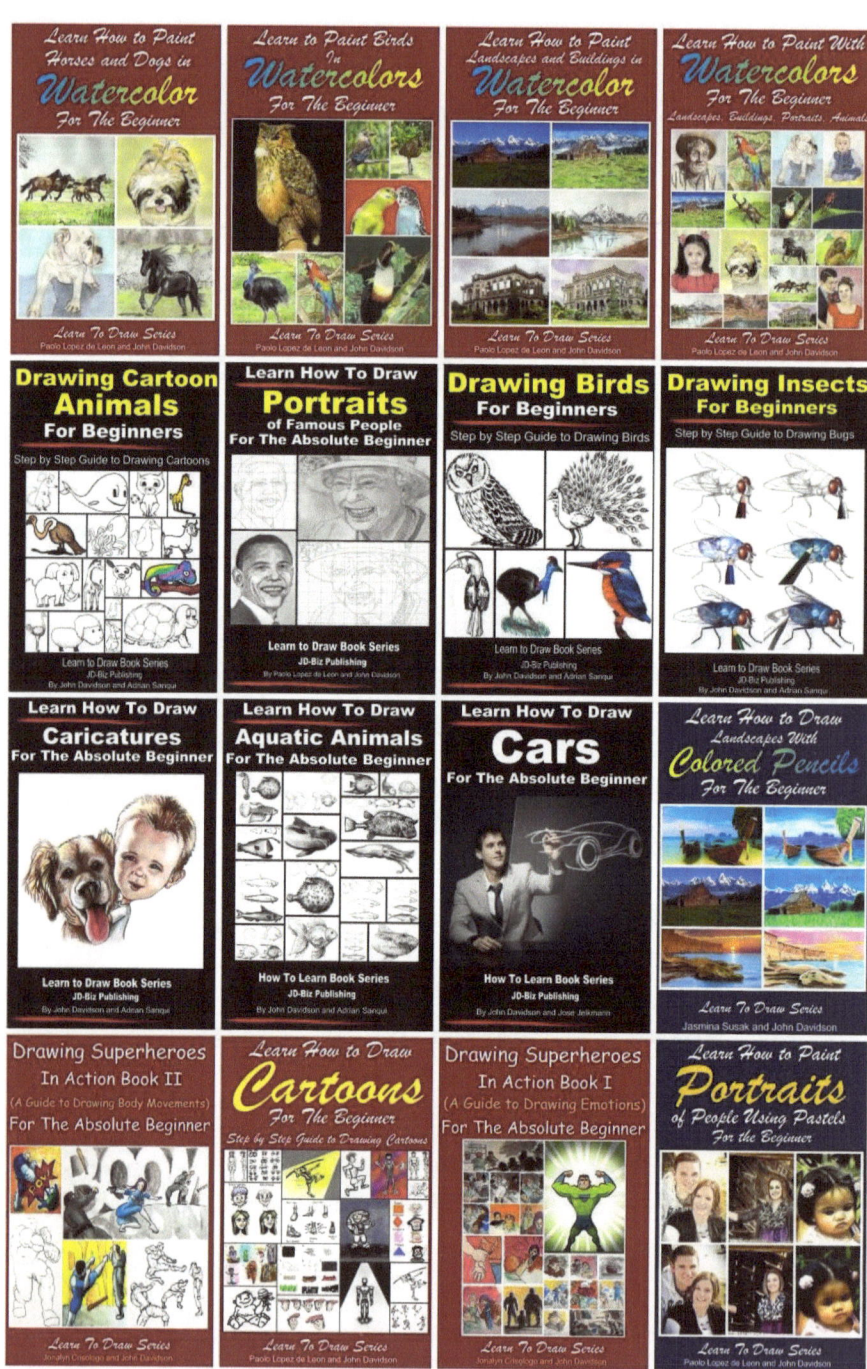

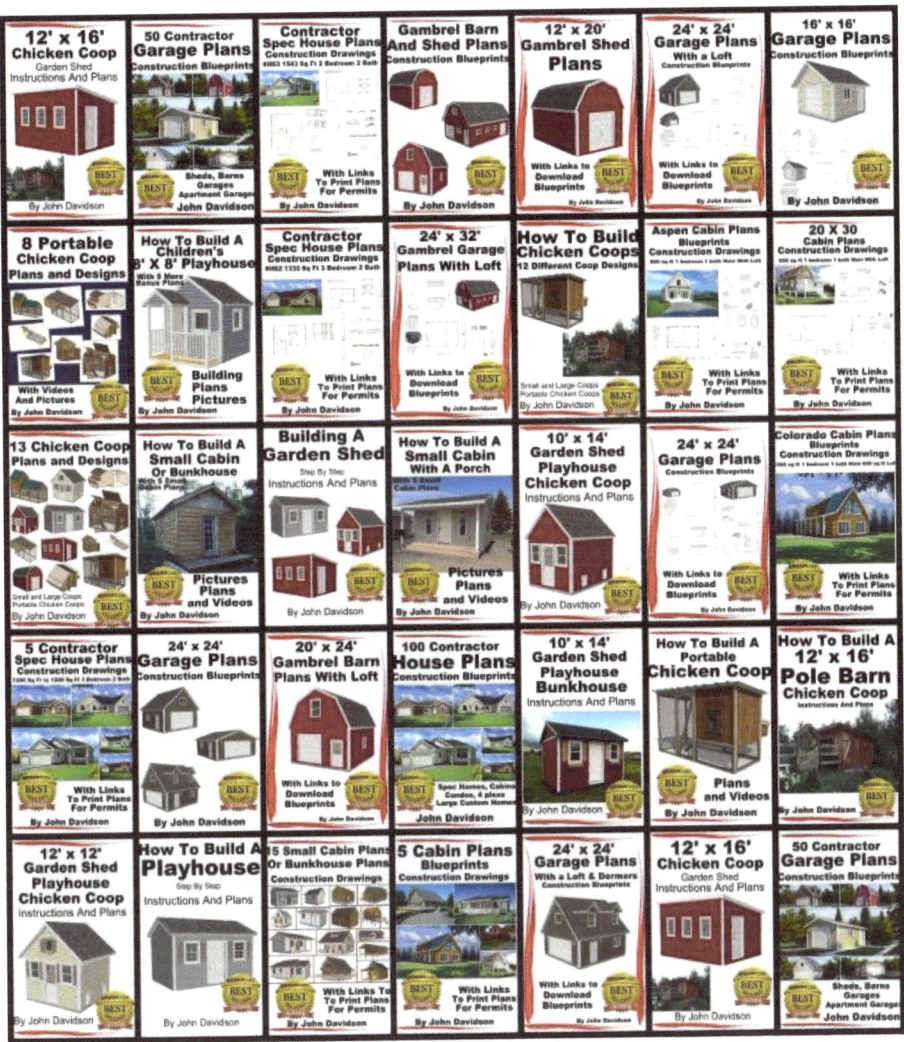

Entrepreneur Book Series

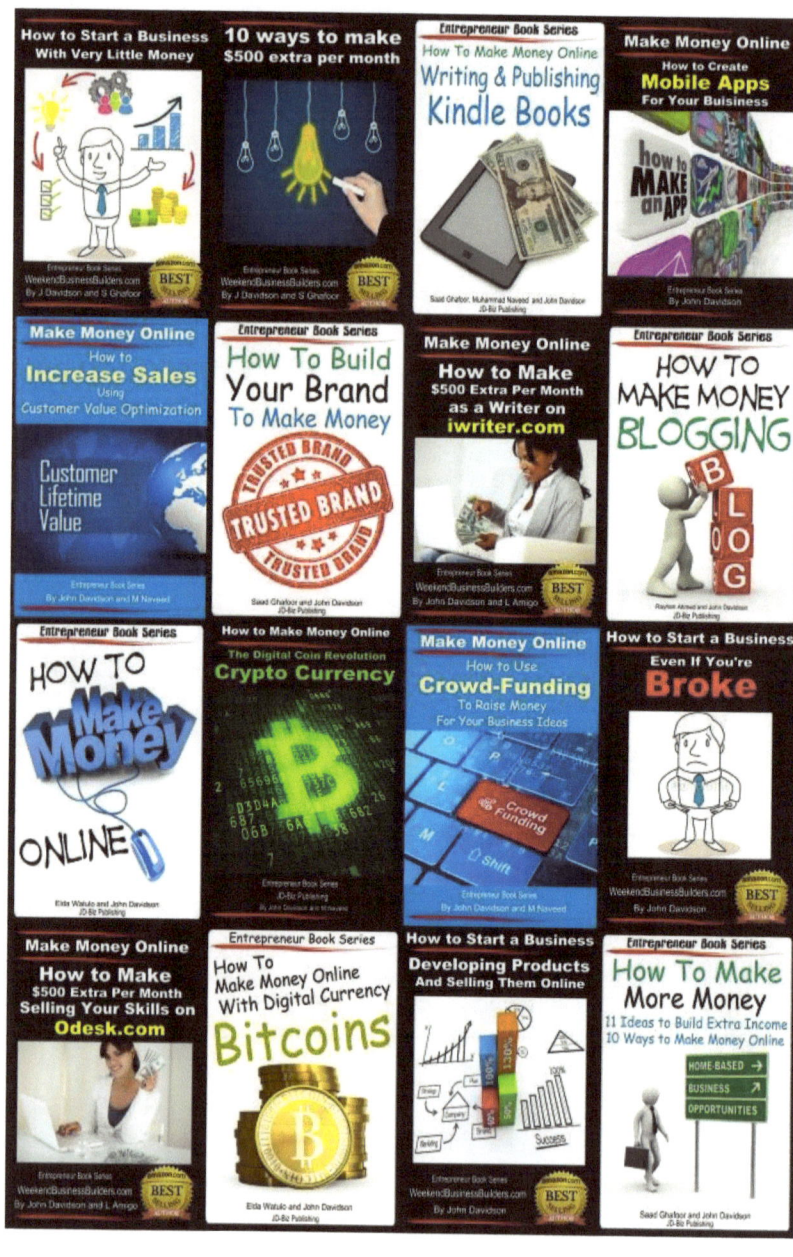

Our books are available at

1. Amazon.com

2. Barnes and Noble

3. Itunes

4. Kobo

5. Smashwords

6. Google Play Books

Download Free Books!

http://MendonCottageBooks.com

Publisher

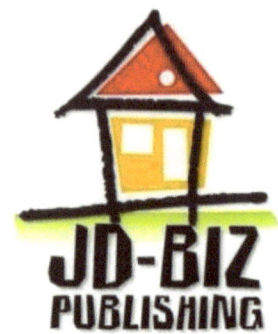

JD-Biz Corp

P O Box 374

Mendon, Utah 84325

http://www.jd-biz.com/

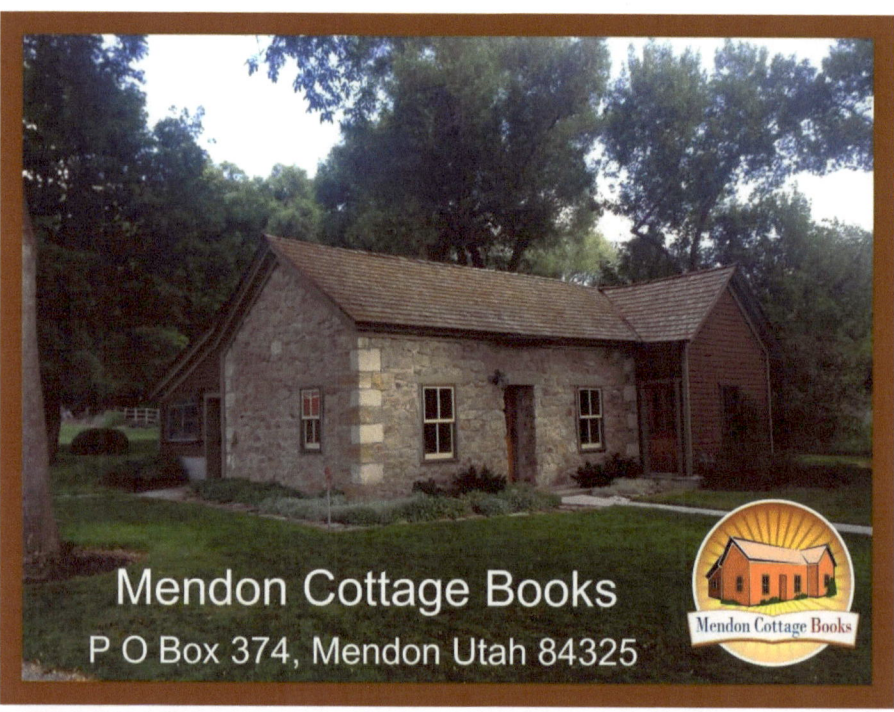

Mendon Cottage Books

P O Box 374, Mendon Utah 84325

www.ingramcontent.com/pod-product-compliance
Lightning Source LLC
Chambersburg PA
CBHW040746010626
45792CB00027B/302